HIIT

The Fastest Way to Get Ripped
and Maximize Your Workout

By Devon Samson

Published in Canada

© Copyright 2015 – Devon Samson

ISBN-13: 978-1514230015
ISBN-10: 1514230011

Table of Contents

Introduction

Read any fitness magazine, blog, or other health related article claiming to help you lose weight or possibly rev the ole' sex drive up again and you are quite literally bound to come across the word *cardio*. Cardio, in its literal definition, is any form of activity or exercise which will challenge and therefore strengthen the capabilities and efficiencies of the body's cardiovascular system (that which circulates blood enriched with oxygen and nutrients to all of your organs, muscles, and ahem...favorite extremities, for those unaware). In the fitness and wellness industry however, nothing of any sort is clear cut.

Numerous opinions abound on the various methods of which cardio can be performed, and their overall effectiveness in comparison to one another. One such topic of debate is the newly rising to popularity method of High Intensity Interval Training (or HIIT, to save that lazy tongue of yours the time). Within this short eBook that you so luckily happen to be reading, the basics, theory, and science of HIIT will be laid out on a platter for you.

What is HIIT Devon?

That's a great question, and I'm glad even though you never asked. You don't need to be a rocket scientist to understand the basis of high intensity interval training. This isn't even high school geometry level stuff we're dealing with here. For a better comprehension of this style of training, we'll start by going through the name bit by bit much like an elementary teacher would with a child having trouble sounding out a word. Begin with the words - *high intensity*. Obviously, this training will include a level of intensity that is above your average output and will require a large demand of oxygen. The second part - *interval training*. No secrets here, you'll be working with intervals (periods of time).

So, what do we get when we put the words together and have *High Intensity Interval Training*? HIIT in its simplistic definition is a style of cardio which incorporates a mixture of extremely high intensity exercise for short bursts of time with periods of low intensity exercise filling the gaps between those short bursts. For a very straight forward example, think of sprinting hard for 30 seconds, and then slowly jogging for 45 seconds. The process is then repeated as many times as desired. This my friend, is HIIT.

Why Does HIIT Work So Well?

Without spoiling all the fun things we'll talk about in Part 2 of this Ebook, there are a host of reasons that High Intensity Interval Training is extremely effective. HIIT increases the efficiency of your anaerobic threshold (in simple terms, the method by which your body burns stored energy without the presence of oxygen), increases the body's maximal oxygen uptake, and can even release certain feel-good hormones that can make working out even more enjoyable than it already is. Cutting edge stuff, ladies and gents.

Who is HIIT For?

To the point, anyone can perform HIIT cardio and reap the benefits. With its fat burning and heart strengthening benefits, High Intensity Interval Training makes a good candidate for any trainee's weekly routine or split. For beginners, HIIT eliminates the need for long periods of daily steady-state cardio that could possibly be a deterrent to continuing on with their training. Athletes will find HIIT to be a vital part of their routines as it builds explosiveness and trains them for sport related situations that could call upon the short bursts of intensity that this style of training entails.

Even the largest or strongest of weight trainees can use HIIT to strip fat levels and "shred up" following an extended bulking period, or possibly add to their strength potential because weight lifting is an anaerobic metabolic pathway similar to HIIT. Before you make a decision on adding HIIT into your training regimen, it's important that you carefully compare and consider it against another time-tested method...steady-state cardio.

Chapter 1:
HIIT vs Steady State

Congratulations, you've weathered all four pages of the introduction and made it to the meat and potatoes of this eBook. Pat yourself on the back, grab a protein shake, kick back, and get educated.

Contest 1: Exercise Enjoyment

No one puts their full effort into something they don't enjoy. It's like your father signing you up for that baseball/softball team as a kid and you sucking the joint out because you had absolutely no desire to play other than the fact you were forced. It may be a far-fetched comparison, but it definitely gets the point across. Are you more likely to give your all at something you enjoy and are passionate about, or something you dread doing?

It's a no-brainer. However, the line here between High Intensity Interval Training and Steady State is very much in the eye of the beholder. There are obvious advantages for both versions of cardio pertaining to the "exercise enjoyment" factor. HIIT employs a very challenging and fast-paced training style that seems to beckon to some people. This fast-paced style eliminates the traditional view of monotony usually associated with performing cardiovascular exercise. On the other end of the spectrum, steady-state cardio is often long drawn out and relatively non-adrenaline triggering. If you get excited to walk on the treadmill and stare at the same wall for an hour straight until you burn your target calories, then more power to you. However, steady state doesn't necessarily mean boring. Many opt to jog along trails or other picturesque scenery and swear by their methods. For this reason, it would be unfair to say that either style is superior to the other in deriving enjoyment from performing.

Contest 2: Exercise Duration

It is here that we start to see a divergence in the two methods. Steady State cardio is just what it says...steady. This steadiness means that the exerciser will be working at about 60-70% of their maximal effort over a period of usually between 30 minutes and upwards of past an hour. For those who have that kind of time, exercise duration won't be a factor in choosing HIIT over Steady State cardio. HIIT on the other hand is much different. Due to its nature of working extremely hard for brief periods of time in a trainee's 90-100% maximal effort range, the workouts are considerably shorter and more condensed. How short? Some can be as short as only 4 minutes, but none should be brushing more than the 30 minute mark. If saving time is in your top priorities, HIIT cardio definitely takes the cake in comparison to long periods of Steady State.

Contest 3: HIIT or Steady State for Weight Loss and Fat Burning Capacity?

In the fitness game, it seems that besides a massive pair of arms, everyone is after *weight loss*. Had too many Twinkies over the years? *Weight Loss.* Wife bugging you about that beer belly? *Weight Loss.* Just have a baby and need to trim up a bit? *Weight Loss.* So it is no surprise that this question is one of the most popular in the debate between High Intensity Interval Training and Steady State Cardio. To jump right in, we'll examine the capacities of Steady State. Steady State cardio as you may have picked up by now is highly aerobic (we'll cover this very soon, but for right now just know that it requires a constant supply of oxygen).

Make no mistake, while you are performing this type of low intensity cardiovascular exercise, your body is burning calories proportional to the rate at which you are capable of steadily moving (the pace at which you are jogging for that extended period of time). However, when your session ends, this calorie-burning party is over. The body performs homeostasis to return its internal balance and temperature, and the effects are over until your next session. Some exercise experts still promote steady state as superior for fat loss as it is believed fatty acid utilization starts to occur only after roughly 30 minutes of training. HIIT blatantly contradicts this theory. High intensity workouts demand extreme levels of oxygen during the session, creating shortage.

This is the vital fact which makes HIIT more effective for fat and weight loss. It is due to this shortage that the body requires more oxygen during recovery and instills an "After burn" effect referred to as Excess Post Exercise Oxygen Consumption (EPOC, nobody knows what happened to the second E so don't ask about it). EPOC is the reason HIIT will not only burn calories and fat DURING exercise, but up to 48 hours AFTER the workout has finished. Say hello to increased metabolism...that's a pretty awesome thing.

Contest 4: Increasing the Anaerobic Threshold

It's time for a biology lesson, children. Gather around Uncle Devon. Within each little cell of our bodies, are *organelles* which perform specific cell functions. You can think of these as microscopic organs, except they belong to cells. The name of the organelles which provide energy for the cell are called the *mitochondria*. The mitochondria go through a process called cellular respiration (the opposite of photosynthesis, for those curious) to produce energy for the cell. There are two pathways for cellular respiration whose names have already been mentioned briefly throughout the eBook: Aerobic and Anaerobic Respiration. In aerobic respiration, glucose (the stuff in carbohydrates) enters the cytoplasm of the cell and creates a substance called *pyruvate* which then enters the mitochondria.

With a supply of oxygen, the mitochondria can then produce Adenosine Triphosphate (ATP), the compound responsible for releasing energy on a cellular level. Since steady state cardio is over a long duration of time it demands a continuous flow of oxygen, making it highly aerobic. However, oxygen is not always readily available for cells. When oxygen is not readily available to convert glucose into ATP molecules, anaerobic respiration occurs. In humans, this process is known as *lactate fermentation.*

The ins-and-outs of lactate fermentation and how it produces ATP is highly complicated, but the key factor to remember is that it produces *lactic acid*. Unless you've never exercised or done anything moderately strenuous in your lifetime, you know the burning feeling in your muscles from the build-up of lactic acid. If not, stand up and do some calf raises right now until you feeling a searing sensation just above your achilles.

That's lactic acid build-up. HIIT cardio demands quick bursts of power from the muscular and cardiovascular (also technically muscular) systems that create a shortage of oxygen in the body. To meet the physical challenge, the body switches over into anaerobic respiration. HIIT cardio obviously therefore improves the anaerobic threshold much better than aerobic exercise, meaning that you will be able to utilize this advantageous system of power for longer periods of time and more efficiently.

Contest 5: Beta-Endorphin Release

Beta-Endorphins are the chemical compounds that the body releases in order to minimize pain, and have been shown in studies to be as effective as morphine. Endorphins such as these are released in almost all types of exercise, and this is theorized to be the reason why so many people feel extremely happy or content (despite being tired) following a workout. However, the *type* of exercise performed affects the amount of beta endorphin released into the bloodstream. It has been shown in studies that High Intensity Interval Training causes beta endorphin levels to rise in proportion to the extent of lactate concentration (the amount of lactic acid building up in the working muscles).

Beta endorphin levels will peak when a trainee is at the point of or exceeds their personal anaerobic threshold, as was discussed in the last section. In studies done on steady-state exercise performed on an endurance level, beta-endorphin level concentration in the blood is not shown to rise until the 1 hour mark has been surpassed, and may rise incrementally following that. In this case, HIIT cardio trumps steady-state for quick beta-endorphin release and possibly in comparison for the AMOUNT released as well.

Contest 6: VO$_2$ Max

In exercise science, VO$_2$ Max refers to the maximal uptake of oxygen that an individual can use. This is specifically measured by milligrams per kilogram of body weight per minute. It had been traditionally thought by many that steady-state endurance exercise was the most effective way to increase the efficiency of a person's maximal oxygen uptake. Despite this, a more recent examination in various experiments and studies has shown that HIIT is superior in triggering physiological adaptations that enhance an individual's VO$_2$ Max, as well as skeletal muscle cells' mitochondrial enzyme production (increases the efficiency of the energy output of muscle cells).

Contest 7: Athletic Performance

Let's look at this one very logically. In most athletic sports and contests, unless you are a marathon runner that is, your body is required to have quick bursts of speed, power, and agility. Therefore, athletes will be extremely dependent on the strength of their anaerobic system. As we've learned so far, the very best way to strengthen the effectiveness of the anaerobic system is through High Intensity Interval Training. This is not to say though, that low intensity endurance training is completely useless for athletic performance.

The anaerobic and aerobic systems work in tandem with one another, with each doing more work than the other depending on the situation. In the case of an athletic event, as the duration continues to drag on, the phosphocreatine levels within muscle cells will begin to dwindle and the anaerobic system inside the mitochondria will be forced to switch back over to glycolysis (aerobic system). This is why teams who have clearly done more long distance running in practice hours will be able to outlast teams who have done less near the end of the game. In essence, the most strategic plan for all serious athletes is to make time for BOTH types of cardiovascular training in their workout regimen.

HIIT vs. Steady State Summary

As we can see from the comparisons above, HIIT does mainly reign supreme in production of beta endorphins, improving the body's maximal oxygen uptake capacity, potential for fat loss, shorter exercise duration, and increasing the body's' anaerobic threshold. This is not to say that in any shape or form HIIT can clear-cut be labeled "better" than steady-state endurance training. Some trainees will prefer one or the other for personal reasons. There is in my mind no harm in pursuing both methods of training for the best results.

Chapter 2:
HIIT Implementation

The Required HIIT Intensity

High Intensity Interval Training is called High Intensity Interval Training for a reason. Assuming that a HIIT workout is easier than a steady-state workout based on the fact that it is much shorter is a very large mistake. During the short bursts of the workout, you should be giving absolutely everything you have in the tank. Your heart rate, if measured, would be between 90-100% of its maximum. Even within the rest or "low intensity periods" between those short bursts, your heart rate should not fall below 55-60% of its maximum. This will challenge the body's anaerobic system and cause a metabolic disturbance that will have the body burning calories for up to 48 hours afterwards.

HIIT Frequency

High Intensity Interval Training is extremely taxing on the cardiovascular, muscular, and central nervous system. It's for this reason that it is recommended that AT MOST it be performed 4 days of the week. This protocol is reserved for a trainee who performs no other types of training during his or her weekly regimen. HIIT frequency should be reduced for individuals who regularly train with weights to ensure proper muscle recovery. In the case of a weight training athlete looking to reduce fat or increase cardiovascular health, I prescribe reducing HIIT sessions to three times a week, and performing steady-state on two separate days.

Modes and Getting the Most Out Of HIIT

Contrary to popular belief, HIIT doesn't have to be the traditional grueling set of sprints or bouts of speed on the elliptical machine (although it can be). Any form of exercise that incorporates periods of high intensity separated with periods of low intensity is considered HIIT. HIIT can be worked in while swimming, rowing, performing bodybuilding circuits, or if you really want to go down that route...crossfit. Weapons of choice include kettlebells, dumbbells, exercise balls, atlas stones, sledgehammers, and wheelbarrows (for distance wheeling).

HIIT as stated before is an extremely simple concept. As long as you are working at the required intensity and with indomitable commitment, you are going to see results. The results you want are only limited by what you desire. Tailoring the style of HIIT (whether it is strictly cardio, bodybuilding circuit, swimming, rowing, or Crossfit) to your own personal goals is what really matters in getting the most out of your High Intensity Interval Training.

Nutrition While On HIIT

Nutrition is a branching topic, again centered around an individual's personal goals. The main purpose of HIIT for most trainees will inevitably be for fat loss. Losing fat is not a complicated process, and is often blurred in difficulty by the media and by unmotivated people who are unsuccessful in doing it. If your goal is to lose fat while utilizing HIIT, first calculate your daily weight maintenance calories.

From here, it as simple as consuming 250 calories *less* per day. Make 50% of those calories proteins, 25% of them carbs, and 25% of them fats. That's it. HIIT will also do you the favor of burning *more* calories beyond the calories that you cut in that method. For pre-HIIT workout nutrition, consume a light carbohydrate and protein source about an hour before hand. A whole banana with 2 tbsp. of peanut butter should do the trick, but obviously your carbohydrate and protein sources can be swapped out for your own preferences.

Pitfalls of HIIT

Although High Intensity Interval Training is in my opinion (as well as countless others) an invaluable tool in losing fat and improving cardiovascular health, it is in all truthfulness not suited for all trainees. HIIT is fast-paced and strenuous, which leads to a higher risk of injury. Depending on body position during exercise, blood can pool in the lower extremities or dizziness can onset.

In addition, attempting to push too hard as a beginner without first progressing can lead to overly excessive muscle soreness or in the worst case, rhabdomyolysis (damaged muscle fibers breaking off and entering the bloodstream, causing poisoning of the kidneys). Practice common sense and see a doctor to diagnose any possible diseases or limitations before attempting to begin any HIIT workouts or programs.

Sample HIIT Workouts

If you've been reading this short eBook and been sold on the idea of using HIIT and reaping the benefits, then you're in luck. Here is a compilation of a few of my personally chosen HIIT workout samples for you to try out for yourself. From these templates, you can even begin to design your own personally-made routines. Is that eagerness I sense?

FIVE Beginner-Level Workouts

#1: Treadmill/Elliptical Classic HIIT

(This should take roughly 10 minutes to perform. This will not include the recommended 3 minutes of light jogging to warm up beforehand, or the 3 minutes of light jogging to cool down after the workout)

Perform 20 seconds of intense speed

Perform 40 seconds of recovery jogging.

Repeat this process 10 times.

#2: Beginner – Friendly 10 Minute Bodyweight HIIT Workout

Perform each exercise at high intensity for 45 seconds followed by 15 seconds of rest. Then move onto the next exercise. Once through the circuit, rest two minutes and repeat 4 times.

Mountain Climbers
Push-Ups
Air-Squats
Crunches
Burpees (Squat Thrusts)
Plank
Jump Squats
Jumping Jacks
High Knees
Lunges

#3: Simple Outdoor Fat Scorcher

Find a small sized hill, an area to do push-ups at the top of this hill, and a spot to perform low-intensity jumping jacks at the bottom.

Sprint as hard as possible up the hill
Upon reaching the top of the hill, perform 15 push-ups.Jog down the hill, and perform low-intensity (meaning don't be going insanely fast) jumping jacks for 1 minute at the bottom.
Repeat this process 10 times.

#4: 20 Minute Calorie Burner

During this workout, you will perform five different movements. For 45 seconds you will attempt to perform as many reps as possible, and then rest 15 seconds before moving onto the next exercise and repeating. There will be 3 rounds of this, and 1 minute rest between each round.

Push-ups (modified if necessary) - 45 seconds
Rest - 15 seconds
Air Squats - 45 seconds
Rest - 15 seconds
Butt Kicks - 45 seconds
Rest - 15 seconds
Tricep Dips - 45 seconds
Rest - 15 seconds
Side Lunges - 45 seconds
Rest one minute and repeat the round

#5: Butt – Toner

This is one of the most simple HIIT workouts out there and will help the ladies (and who knows, maybe guys too) get the glutes and thighs that both they and the opposite sex desire. There will be a total of five rounds, with no rest between these rounds. Get to it.

10 squat jumps

30 second wall-sit

20 Forward Lunges (10 for each leg)

30 second wall-sit

Repeat

FIVE Intermediate-Level Workouts

#1: Jump Rope Oriented HIIT Workout

50 reps of Jump Roping
1o push-ups
10 Burpees
20 High Knees
50 reps of Jump Roping
10 squat jumps
10 reverse lunges (each leg)
10 burpees
50 reps of Jump Roping
20 crunches
10 flutter kicks

#2: *Stadium Runner Workout*

It's time to head to your local high school football stadium and hit the bleachers. For this simple yet challenging workout, you will begin by sprinting full-steam up the stairs until reaching the top. At the top of the bleachers, you will then attempt to hold a plank for the MAXIMUM amount of time possible. You will have 30 seconds to rest before jogging back down the bleachers and immediately sprinting back up to begin the next round.

Bleacher Sprint
Max-Duration Plank Hold
30 second Rest
Jog down the bleachers
Repeat.

#3: Burpee Warfare

Burpees have been a longtime conditioning favorite of American football coaches, and with good reason. The exercise entails going from a standing position, to flat on your face, to standing again, and is extremely demanding on the body's aerobic AND anaerobic fitness level. It is recommended you perform this routine on soft running track or in grass so you can stop where you are jogging to complete the burpees.

1 Minute - Perform as many burpees as possible

1 Minute : Light jog at approximately 60% of your full effort

Repeat this process 10 times

#4: Leapfrog HIIT Workout

Perform the following exercises for two rounds, with the objective of completing these two rounds in the shortest amount of time possible.

10 Squat Jumps

20 Plyo (Jumping) Push-Ups

30 Forward Lunges (15 to each leg)

40 Box Jumps

50 Jump Rope Repetitions

Repeat.

TIP: To make plyo push-ups easier, simply perform them as a regular push-up, on an incline, or on your knees. For more of a challenge, attempt to clap your hands together mid-air as your propel yourself from the ground using your chest and triceps.

#5: 7 Minutes to Rock Hard Abs

Weighted Plank - 1 Minute

Perform as many Spiderman Push-Ups as possible in 1 Minute

30 second rest

Perform as many lying V-Ups as possible in 1 Minute

Perform as many Sit-Ups as possible in 1 Minute

30 second rest

Perform as many Seated Leg Tucks as possible in 1 Minute

Perform as many Flutter Kicks as possible in 1 Minute

FIVE Advanced-Level Workouts

#1: Bodybuilding Style HIIT: Chest and Back

Bench Press - 1o sets of 10 reps - use 50% maximum weight - 30 second rests

Dumbbell Incline Press - 3 sets of 10 reps - 45 seconds rest

Dumbbell Decline Press - 3 sets of 15 reps - 30 second rests

Cable Crossovers - 3 sets of 15 reps - 30 second rests

Wide Grip Lat Pulldown - 10 sets of 10 reps - use 50% maximum weight - 30 second rests

Barbell Bent Over Row - 3 sets of 10 reps - 45 second rests

Straight-Arm Pulldown - 3 sets of 15 reps - 30 second rests

Weighted Hyperextensions - 3 sets of 15 reps - 30 second rests

#2: HIIT Swimming "Ladder" Workout

Warm-up for 5-10 minutes with low-impact cardio exercise such as jogging.

For the following intervals, rest 10-30 seconds between swimming legs depending on your fitness level.

Freestyle stroke 150 meters at a slow pace

Freestyle stroke 120 meters at a medium pace

Freestyle stroke 100 meters at a fast (sprint) pace

Freestyle 120 meters at a medium pace

Freestyle stroke 150 meters at slow pace

Perform a light 5-10 minute cool down to conclude the workout.

#3: Pulling Power HIIT

Next to squats, the barbell deadlift is heralded as the king of all exercises. There is nothing quite as primal as ripping a heavy weight off the ground. If you're a caveman and a rock is blocking the entrance to your cave, what are you going to do? You're going to deadlift that bad boy out of the way. Combine deadlifts with HIIT and you have a recipe for bad-assery.

Perform the following circuit as many times as possible in 10 minutes.

Deadlifts - 10 reps with 65% of 1 rep-max weight
Box Jumps - 10 reps
Repeat.

#4: Boxer HIIT

Fighters are some of the most well-conditioned and shredded athletes on the planet. This workout mimics their training and will help you sculpt the physique you've been after. You will need a heavy punching bag and gloves. Aim to perform 3 rounds in the quickest amount of time possible.

20 jabs (each hand)

20 knee jabs (each knee)

40 dumbbell punches (step away from the bag and perform air-punches grasping light dumbbells. Each hand will do 20 reps)

50 reps of Jump Rope

Repeat

#5: Death Grip HIIT

Grip strength will aid in all facets of life. From carrying those 5 extra bags of groceries inside to avoid another trip, hoisting those bags of cement to the backyard to start your patio, and other...extracurricular activities...grip strength will play a large role. This workout will ramp up the fat-burning benefits due to its multiple multi-joint movements and extremely high-intensity. Are you up to it? Perform the following circuit for 5 rounds in the quickest amount of time possible.

Rowing Machine - 500 Meters at 80% effort (Alternative: 100 Yard Dumbbell Farmer's Walk - use challenging weights)

Barbell Power Cleans - 10 reps

10 Pull-Ups

Repeat.

#5: HIIT Leg Workout From Hell

Leg training has a legendary reputation for being as brutal as they come. In this case, we'll be going beyond brutal. This workout will be downright nasty, painful, and gut-wrenching. But you cannot gain without sacrifice. This workout will build large, veiny, striated quads and hamstrings while at the same time burning insane amounts of calories and fat. You will be performing two rounds, and if you've challenged yourself correctly by the end, you won't have the energy to do any more than that. Or to drag yourself back to your car. Perform the following circuit while resting only when indicated.

Barbell Back Squats - 15 reps

Leg Press - 6 reps (very heavy weight)

Rest 30 seconds

Leg Extensions - 20 reps (on last round, perform a triple-dropset upon reaching 20 reps)

Dumbbell Stiff-Legged Deadlifts - 10 reps

Rest 2 minutes

Repeat

NOTE: You may perform calf exercises of your choice following the routine if desired.

Chapter 3:
HIIT Myths

HIIT appears to be the perfect solution for weight loss, muscle gain and improved stamina. However, with all the good and bad claims relating to high intensity training, it can be confusing. Below are the common myths associated with HIIT:

1. HIIT should be done daily

HIIT should only be done twice or three times a week, to allow your muscles to rest and regenerate. Daily intense workouts are not practical, as it requires a high level of energy and concentration, which people don't normally have. Also, HIIT causes muscle pain after the workout and it takes one to two days for the body to recover.

HIIT is beneficial for people who don't abuse their body and workout program. You need to read your own body and adjust accordingly to avoid overtraining and associated injuries.

2. HIIT is limited to sprinting and sprinters

HIIT can be done indoors or outdoors. It is also not limited to sprinting or jogging alone. Though sprinting is commonly used in many HIIT programs, there are a lot of other exercises being used too. These are, jumping jacks, high knees, mountain climbers, burpees, and walking to name a few.

It is not only beneficial for sprinters, but for athletes or people who want to increase their stamina and increase metabolism.

3. HIIT follows strict eating patterns

HIIT does not follow a scheduled eating plan. There are no required pre or post intense training meals. A person can eat anytime that is convenient to him/her. But people who undergo HIIT are advised to eat healthy carbohydrates and natural sugars.

High intensity trainers are given advice to take protein shakes, smoothies or fruit & vegetable juices for added nutrition.

Chapter 4:
The Importance of
Metabolism

All living organisms need metabolism in order to sustain life. This is the mechanism wherein chemical reactions in the body maintain the existing state of cells and organs. This biochemical process involves a complex structure of hormones and enzymes in the body. It affects how we burn the foods we eat and how these foods turn into energy. Simply put, it is our body's way to burn up the calories we used up by eating. It is the rate at which the body processes foods. For one to increase it, it is important to understand more about metabolism.

Metabolism has two different categories: catabolism and anabolism. Catabolism is the breaking down of molecules in order to obtain energy. It provides the energy your body needs for physical activities. Examples of classic catabolic hormones found in the body are cortisol, glucagon, adrenaline, and cytokines. The other one, anabolism, is the synthesis of compounds needed by our cells. Our bodies have anabolic hormones: the growth hormone, insulin, testosterone, estrogen, and other insulin-like growth hormones.

In layman's term, these two divisions have something to do with an individual's diet. But really, is it fair to put the blame on metabolism that some people find it hard to shed some pounds? In effect, these things play a substantial role in a person's body weight because our body mass is just the result of catabolism minus anabolism. Calories consumed minus calories burned equals your current weight.

Because of our unique bodies, each of us was born with a distinct metabolic rate. Aside from hormone levels and sleep, metabolic rate is another factor affecting one's weight. Once we reach 40, our metabolisms decrease at least five percent every 10 years. Though it changes only every decade, it does not mean that your metabolic rate is the same as last year. If you have a higher metabolism today, there's no guarantee that it will be the same in the next years to come as metabolism slows down when people age.

Your metabolic rate is determined by two things. First is the amount of mitochondria you have. It can be found inside your muscle cells. This little "furnace" inside your cells takes in calories from the food you consume. Second is how capable your mitochondria is at burning calories. That can be based on your lifestyle or involvement with physical activities.

Your basal metabolic rate makes up a great fraction of total calories burned. If you want to measure your metabolic rate, then you can check out metabolism calculators over the internet. These days, many health and fitness websites offer basal metabolic rate calculators. All you have to do is state your gender, age, height, weight, and activity level. There are four kinds of activity levels— inactive, lightly inactive, moderately active, very active, and extremely active.

Inactive activity level means little or no exercise at all. Lightly inactive means you only do light exercises once or thrice a week. Moderately active is if you do moderate exercises or sports three to five times a week. Very active means you engage in hard sports six to seven days a week. Lastly, extremely active ones are those who do very hard exercises every day. If you train twice a day or do a physical job, then it can also fall under the extremely active level.

Given all the information to calculate your basal metabolic rate, you will learn the amount of calories you should burn each day. But it is not just your basal metabolic rate that you can evaluate. You can also estimate your resting metabolic rate (RMR) to know how many calories you will burn if you were to do nothing but rest for 24 hours. These two are often used conversely but they still have slight differences. The basal metabolic rate measurement is usually taken in stricter conditions than RMR. Either way, these two measurements will help you comprehend how many calories your body needs in order to function well.

To estimate for your RMR, just add your weight in kilograms and your height in centimeters. Then subtract it to the sum of your age in years and gender. For gender, use one if you are a male and use zero if you are a female. Like BMR, you can also compute for your RMR on health and fitness websites online.

In addition, there are three basic strategies to speed up your metabolic rate. One is to build more mitochondria. Second is to make those mitochondria burn calories as quickly as possible. Third is to make sure that one's thyroid is not cooling one's mitochondria down. Thyroid regulates the rate at which the mitochondria burn calories.

Once again, every individual was born with a unique metabolism. But whatever condition, age or gender you have right now, it is likely for you to shed some pounds by boosting your metabolism.

Chapter 5:
Benefits of Increased Metabolism

Increasing one's metabolic rate can help exhaust more weight minus cutting more calories. Unfortunately, only a few are blessed with a fast metabolism. But there are various ways to increase it. Before coming up with the steps, it is helpful to know its benefits first. Aside from letting you drop some pounds effortlessly, increasing your metabolic rate can help your body burn calories faster than the average.

If you want to increase your metabolic rate, then the first thing you have to do is understand metabolism. If you have a faster metabolism compared to other people, then you will be able to lose more weight even if you share the same weight, diet, and activity level.

One more thing you have to consider are the factors affecting your metabolism. There are some which you cannot change or control like aging, gender, and heredity. After the age of 40, expect your metabolic rate to drop as your muscle mass also fairly decreases. If you're a man, then you normally burn more calories quicker than the opposite gender because men have more muscle tissue. Regarding genes, it is likely for anyone to inherit faster metabolic rates from previous generations.

Aside from these, there are other factors you have to think about such as weight and thyroid disorders. Since muscle is more compressed, it contributes more than fat per unit mass. Meanwhile, there are two types of thyroid disorders. First is hypothyroidism, which means underactive thyroid gland. Second is hyperthyroidism or overactive thyroid gland. These conditions can either rev up or slow down one's metabolism.

You learned about estimating your BMR and RMR in order to identify how much calories your body needs to function. If you are done computing your RMR, then you can now adjust your diet accordingly and build up your metabolism. But if you just want to maintain your weight, then just multiply your RMR by 1.15 and you will discover the extent of your daily consumption. Remember not to exceed your consumption in order to maintain a safe weight. Moreover, you should not have a caloric intake lesser than your calculated RMR.

Conclusion

HIIT Cardio is a mainstream topic in the fitness world. Is High Intensity Interval Training merely a fad born out of ever-changing public trends? It's difficult to say. What we do know, is that HIIT is scientifically backed. Studies reveal its potential to burn fat, save time, release beta endorphins, increase athletic performance, and improve an individual's anaerobic threshold. When compared to its steady-state opposition, HIIT appears to reign supreme in most comparisons. Armed with the knowledge you now possess, you can confidently begin training and benefiting from High Intensity Interval Training today. So get out there and get it, champ.

DISCLAIMER AND/OR LEGAL NOTICES: Every effort has been made to accurately represent this book and it's potential. Results vary with every individual, and your results may or may not be different from those depicted. No promises, guarantees or warranties, whether stated or implied, have been made that you will produce any specific result from this book. Your efforts are individual and unique, and may vary from those shown. Your success depends on your efforts, background and motivation.

The material in this publication is provided for educational and informational purposes only and is not intended as medical advice. The information contained in this book should not be used to diagnose or treat any illness, metabolic disorder, disease or health problem. Always consult your physician or health care provider before beginning any nutrition or exercise program. Use of the programs, advice, and information contained in this book is at the sole choice and risk of the reader.